# VITAMINS & MINERALS

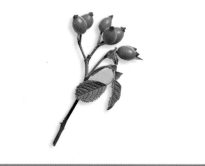

# VITAMINS & MINERALS

## A STEP-BY-STEP
## GUIDE

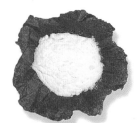

### KAREN SULLIVAN

ELEMENT

SHAFTESBURY, DORSET • ROCKPORT, MASSACHUSETTS • BRISBANE, QUEENSLAND

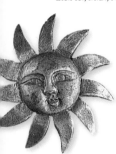

*Dedication*
FOR PUD

Author's acknowledgments
Grateful thanks to Barry Pancham, B.S.,
Lic.Ac., M.B., Ac.A., trace mineral
specialist who
provided advice.

© Element Books
Limited 1997

First published
in Great Britain in
1997 by
ELEMENT BOOKS
LIMITED Shaftesbury,
Dorset, SP7 9BP

Published in the USA in 1997 by
ELEMENT BOOKS INC
PO Box 830, Rockport, MA 01966

Published in Australia in 1997 by
ELEMENT BOOKS LIMITED
for JACARANDA WILEY LIMITED
33 Park Road, Milton, Brisbane 4064

NOTE FROM THE PUBLISHER
Any information given in this book is not
intended to be taken as a replacement for
medical advice. Any person with a
condition requiring medical
attention should consult a
qualified practitioner
or therapist.

*Designed and created with*
*The Bridgewater Book Company Ltd*

ELEMENT BOOKS LIMITED
*Editorial Director* Julia McCutchen
*Managing Editor* Caro Ness
*Production Director* Roger Lane
*Production* Sarah Golden

THE BRIDGEWATER BOOK COMPANY LTD
*Art Director* Peter Bridgewater
*Designers* Andrew Milne, Jane Lanaway
*Page layout* Chris Lanaway, Sue Rose
*Managing Editor* Anne Townley
*Picture Research* Lynda Marshall
*Three dimensional models* Mark Jamieson
*Photography* Ian Parsons, Guy Ryecart
*Illustrations* Andrew Milne, Andrew Kulman
*Text consultants* BOOK CREATION SERVICES LTD
*Series Editor* Karen Sullivan

*Printed and bound in Italy*
*by* Graphicom S.r. l.

British Library Cataloguing in

Publication data available

Library of Congress
Cataloging in Publication
data available

ISBN 1–86204–011–7

*The publishers wish to thank*
*the following for the use of*
*pictures:* e.t. archive: p.8B;
Science Photo Library:
pp.19T, 23TL, 37B, 45T, 47B, 50T; Zefa
Picture Library: pp.9BR, 11TR, 15TR, 24T.

*Special thanks go to:*
Tom Aitken, Carly Evans *for help with*
*photography;* Chris Roberts, Healthcrafts
Ltd, Lewes, Sussex, UK *for supplying vitamins*
*and minerals for photography;* Steamer
Trading Company, Lewes, Sussex, UK *for*
*help with properties.*

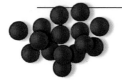

IN A NUTSHELL

VITAMINS & MINERALS

# Contents

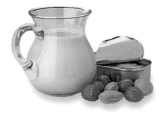

# What are vitamins & minerals?

OUR UNDERSTANDING OF VITAMINS *and minerals, and their role in our body, has improved dramatically over the last decades. We now know that "micronutrition" – or the vitamins, minerals, and other health-giving components of our food – is crucial to life, and that by manipulating our nutritional intake, we can not only ensure good health and address ailments, but also prevent illness and some of the degenerative effects of aging.*

## VITAMINS AND MINERALS

Vitamins are a group of unrelated organic nutrients which are essential to regulate the chemical processes that go on in the body – such as releasing the energy from food, maintaining strong bones, and controlling hormonal activity. Vitamins cannot be made in the body and must be obtained from food, or supplements. Without all the essential vitamins, life cannot be sustained. Carbohydrates, proteins, fats, and vitamins are organic substances, which means that they are all compounds of carbon. We also need nutrients which are not organic. There are two categories of these – those that we need in quantities greater than 100mg per day, and those that are required in quantities less than 100mg per day. The first group are called minerals, the second trace elements; both are necessary for health.

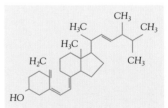

ABOVE *The chemical structures of all vitamins are now known, and they are synthesized in many supplements. This shows the structure of vitamin D.*

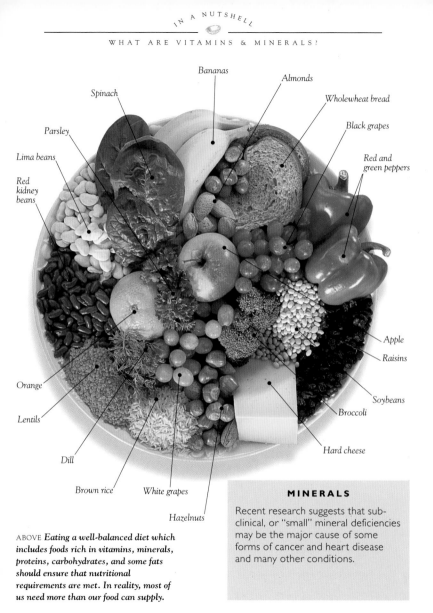

Bananas

Almonds

Spinach

Wholewheat bread

Parsley

Black grapes

Lima beans

Red and green peppers

Red kidney beans

Apple

Raisins

Orange

Soybeans

Lentils

Broccoli

Dill

Hard cheese

Brown rice

White grapes

Hazelnuts

ABOVE *Eating a well-balanced diet which includes foods rich in vitamins, minerals, proteins, carbohydrates, and some fats should ensure that nutritional requirements are met. In reality, most of us need more than our food can supply.*

## MINERALS

Recent research suggests that sub-clinical, or "small" mineral deficiencies may be the major cause of some forms of cancer and heart disease and many other conditions.

# A short history

AWARENESS OF VITAMINS, *minerals, and trace elements is relatively new. Until recently nutrition played a very small role in the conventional treatment of health problems. Today, the stresses of daily living and the assault on our bodies by environmental pollutants have led to an extraordinary array of health problems that has forced an investigation into the relationship between health and the elements of nutrition.*

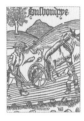

ABOVE *Before intensive farming methods became the norm, the soil was rich with minerals which entered our food.*

## VITAMINS FOR HEALTH

Until the beginning of the twentieth century, we knew very little about nutrition and vitamins were unknown. It was believed that fat, carbohydrates, and proteins, along with some minerals like calcium, were all that was needed to sustain life. Laboratory tests soon proved that theory wrong, and within 30 years, 50 substances were identified as "accessory food factors" which were necessary for living. All 50 factors were given names and numbers, but of those 50, only 13 now remain, for subsequent research made it clear that our bodies could produce some of the necessary components themselves. This explains why there are letters missing in the series of vitamins – i.e., C, D, E, but no F or G.

RIGHT *Before the eighteenth century, a sailor's rations contained no fresh food, causing a deficiency of vitamin C and the illness called "scurvy."*

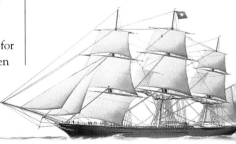

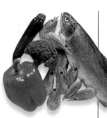

RIGHT *Eating a balanced diet – including 4 to 5 portions of fresh fruit and vegetables each day – should provide us with a diet rich in vitamins and minerals.*

## A HISTORY OF DEFICIENCY

Before the role of vitamins and minerals was understood, there were many deficiency diseases evident in the population; seamen suffered from scurvy, a deficiency of vitamin C, which was caused by a diet of almost exclusively biscuits, salt, meat, and fish. Vitamin C was the subject of the first controlled clinical experiment in recorded medical history. In the 1750s, a British doctor put limes, which are rich in vitamin C, into the diet of a group of sailors and compared this with a second group who received regular rations. The sailors who had a diet rich in vitamin C did not develop scurvy, so citrus fruit became a regular feature in the diets of English sailors – who became known as "limeys."

Sixty years ago there was a widespread incidence of pellagra in South America. Pellagra is characterized by dementia, diarrhea, and dermatitis, and its spread was so rampant that a plague warning was issued. In the end, a deficiency of vitamin B3, niacin, was proved to be the cause of the "plague," and pellagra is now extremely rare in the West.

### DAMAGE TO FOOD

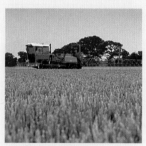

Pollutants and modern methods of farming damage our food and expose us to environmental stresses that place enormous demands on our bodies and rob them of vital nutrients.

# The role of vitamins & minerals

VITAMINS AND MINERALS *and other trace elements work together within the body to ensure that all processes can be carried out. When even one element is missing, the body becomes unbalanced and unable to work at optimum level. Think of your body as a well-oiled machine – when one part gets jammed, nothing works effectively.*

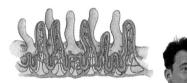

ABOVE **Water-soluble vitamins (the B vitamins and vitamin C) must be taken daily to prevent deficiency.**

*Tissues need a regular supply of water-soluble vitamins*

## HOW VITAMINS & MINERALS WORK

In the body, proteins, carbohydrates, and fats combine with other substances to yield energy and build bones and tissue. These chemical reactions are accelerated by specific vitamins. The vitamins we need are divided into two categories: water-soluble vitamins (the B vitamins and vitamin C) and fat-soluble vitamins (A, D, E, and K). Water-soluble vitamins are not stored in the body and must be taken daily to prevent deficiency. Fat-soluble vitamins can be stored in larger amounts than water-soluble vitamins. The intestine absorbs them, and the lymphatic system carries them to the different parts of the body. Fat-soluble vitamins are involved in maintaining the structure of cell membranes. Excessive intake of fat-soluble vitamins, particularly vitamins A and D, can lead to toxic levels in the body.

There are 18 known minerals required for the maintenance of our bodies. Without minerals, vitamins cannot be assimilated.

Ideally, vitamins and minerals are found in all organic foods, but in reality, processing and other modern methods of food production may deplete them.

## DEFICIENCY SYMPTOMS

Your body will make clear when even small deficiencies are present.

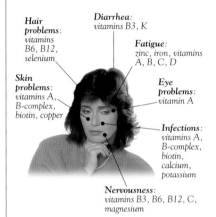

*Hair problems:* vitamins B6, B12, selenium

*Diarrhea:* vitamins B3, K

*Fatigue:* zinc, iron, vitamins A, B, C, D

*Skin problems:* vitamins A, B-complex, biotin, copper

*Eye problems:* vitamin A

*Infections:* vitamins A, B-complex, biotin, calcium, potassium

*Nervousness:* vitamins B3, B6, B12, C, magnesium

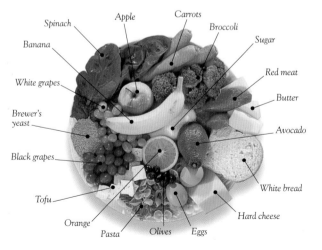

Spinach
Apple
Carrots
Broccoli
Banana
Sugar
White grapes
Red meat
Brewer's yeast
Butter
Black grapes
Avocado
Tofu
Orange
Pasta
Olives
Eggs
Hard cheese
White bread

LEFT *Macronutrients are carbohydrates, fat, and protein, all of which provide energy. Micronutrients are vitamins, minerals, and other minute substances which do not produce energy, but are necessary for the body to release it. Most foods contain macro- and micronutrients.*

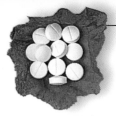

# Treatment

ABOVE **Many people find vitamin tablets are the easiest form in which to take supplements.**

EXCITING DEVELOPMENTS *in the study of micronutrition have meant that more and more of us are taking nutritional supplements. Even healthy diets may no longer have the requisite nutritional elements, and in order to have immune systems that are strong enough to fight off disease and to have optimum levels of energy and mental acuity, we must find these elements elsewhere.*

## SUPPLEMENTS

Supplements should always be taken with care. Never take more than the recommended dosage unless you are under the strict supervision of a nutritionist or practitioner. Some vitamins and minerals can be toxic in excess.

**Vitamin A** can improve eyesight; build resistance to respiratory infections; promote healthy strong bones, hair, skin, teeth, and gums; treat hyperthyroidism and emphysema; treat acne, impetigo, and other skin conditions. Toxic levels can cause hair loss, nausea, vomiting, diarrhea, skin problems, vision problems, rashes, irregular periods, liver enlargement, and birth defects in the babies of women who take vitamin A while pregnant.

**Vitamin B1** (thiamine) can promote growth; treat herpes; relieve post-operative pain; help

RIGHT **Iron is traditionally used to treat some forms of anemia.**

the nervous system and heart to function; improve mental agility and aid digestion. Toxic levels can in rare cases cause tremors, edema, nervousness, palpitations, and allergies.

**Vitamin B6** (pyridoxine) can assimilate protein and fat; work as a diuretic; help prevent nervous and skin problems; alleviate nausea; reduce leg cramps, hand numbness, and muscle spasms. Toxic levels can cause neurological disorders; slight overdoses can cause restlessness at night.

More than half of the population of North America and the UK now take supplements, and contemporary research is in support of their prudent use. We have discovered that the ACE vitamins, along with zinc and selenium, are antioxidants, which can help to prevent heart disease, arthritis, diabetes, and the degenerative processes of aging. Every other vitamin and mineral has a specific function and protective role in the body. Supplements are not a replacement for food, and they cannot be ingested without it. They are no substitute for a poor diet, but they will enhance a good one.

Vitamins and minerals work in conjunction with one another, and megadosing on one can upset the body's balance. A good vitamin and mineral supplement will ensure that you are getting correct amounts.

LEFT *Vitamin E is an antioxidant vitamin and is used to treat many skin conditions, among other things.*

## WHICH SUPPLEMENTS, WHEN?

**Vitamins A, D, E (fat-soluble)** Take regularly with food.

**Iron** On an empty stomach (although it can cause nausea in some cases).

**Calcium** High doses should be taken at night or between meals.

**Zinc** Should be taken with a meal; can cause nausea if taken with insufficient food.

**Vitamin B complex** First thing in the morning for maximum efficiency.

**Vitamin C** Most effective taken with meals and safest at this time if you have an acid-sensitive stomach.

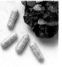

**Magnesium** Can promote sleepiness, so best to take it at night.

**Multivitamins, anti-oxidants** Any time of day is effective and safe – take minerals (except those above) with a drink, such as water.

**Time-release supplements** Take with your main meal.

Try to avoid taking any one vitamin in excess. If you have to take 1,000mg of vitamin C, for example, divide the dose between three meals.

## How and when?

Vitamins and minerals work most effectively when taken evenly throughout the day. The best time for taking most supplements is with meals. Vitamins in particular are organic substances and should be taken with other food and minerals for best absorption. Time-release formulas need to be taken with food, for their nutrients are slowly released over a period of hours. If there is not enough food to slow their passage through the body, they can pass the sites where they are normally absorbed before they've had a chance to release their nutrients. The label on your supplement should advise you of the best time to take it. See the chart on page 13 for tips on taking specific supplements to best effect.

## A PROFESSIONAL APPROACH

Most vitamins and minerals can be safely taken without input from a nutritionist, but if you suffer from chronic health problems or a specific ailment, it is best to seek expert advice. A nutritionist can make sure that any trace deficiencies are corrected, and that you are taking a balanced combination of vitamins and minerals which will work together to make you healthy. Many doctors and complementary practitioners

### WARNING

Children's needs are much lower than adults', and supplements should be given with great care. Read the label to ensure that the product is safe for children and follow the directions carefully.

BELOW *Consult a nutritional therapist if you suffer from long-term illness or you need advice.*

recommend taking certain supplements, since nutrition is the foundation of good health on every level.

## Can treatment be combined with other therapies or drugs?

Strictly speaking, vitamins and minerals are elements of food, and are safe to take with other medication and with complementary treatments. Tell your physician if you are taking supplements and they will advise you if there are contra-indications. Supplements are just that – they supplement a healthy diet – and in moderation they are safe additions to any treatment.

### WARNING

Our needs change in pregnancy. Extra folic acid and iron, and a good multivitamin and mineral supplement, are often suggested.
Do not take vitamin A supplements while pregnant (see page 22).

## TREATMENT PERIOD EFFECTS OVER TIME

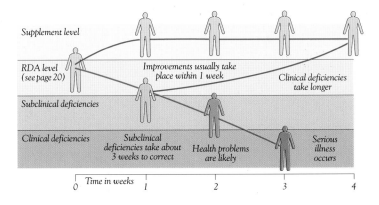

Supplement level

RDA level (see page 20)

Improvements usually take place within 1 week

Clinical deficiencies take longer

Subclinical deficiencies

Clinical deficiencies

Subclinical deficiencies take about 3 weeks to correct

Health problems are likely

Serious illness occurs

Time in weeks

0      1      2      3      4

# Vitamins & minerals in our food

IN WHOLE, ORGANIC FOODS *there should be high levels of vitamins and minerals. Ideally, our nutritional intake should be adequate so that supplementation is kept to a minimum – and that means ensuring that we have a varied, balanced diet.*

## TYPICAL MEALS CONTAINING A BALANCE OF VITAMINS & MINERALS

RIGHT **A varied diet will provide the balance of nutrients required. Vegetarians and vegans have special needs, but the nutritional elements of meat and animal products can be replaced with careful planning.**

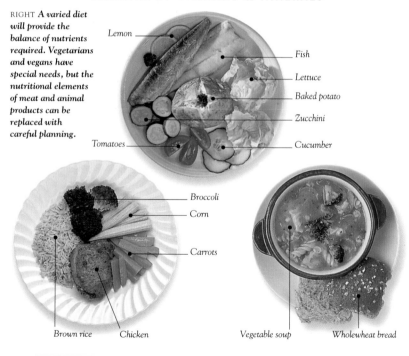

Lemon

Fish

Lettuce

Baked potato

Zucchini

Tomatoes

Cucumber

Broccoli

Corn

Carrots

Brown rice    Chicken

Vegetable soup    Wholewheat bread

## OUR DAILY DIET

Our diet should be made up of complex carbohydrates (5–9 portions per day), fruits and vegetables (4–9 portions), proteins (3–5 portions), and fat (less than 35 percent of our diet is recommended). But eating the right foods doesn't necessarily mean that you are getting enough vitamins and minerals. Remember that refining foods takes out most of the nutritional value.

### Tips for maximum nutrition

• Eat the skins of fruits and vegetables whenever possible.

• Don't cut, wash, or soak fruits and vegetables until you are ready to eat them.

• Eat brown, unpolished rice and whole grains.

• Choose fresh fruit and vegetables first, but remember that nutritional value decreases with age. Frozen is a better option if you aren't going to eat the food immediately.

• Eat raw food whenever possible; if cooking, use as little water as possible.

• Organic food is generally more nutritious.

**FOOD VALUES**

 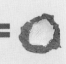

*8mg calcium*

*3.5oz(100g) pears provides only 8mg of calcium, about 1 percent of the recommended daily allowance for women.*

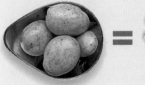

*100mg vitamin C*

*You would need to eat 2.2Ib(1kilo) of potatoes to give you 100mg of vitamin C, the daily requirement now recommended.*

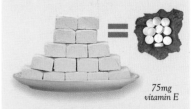

*75mg vitamin E*

*7.7Ib(3.5kilos) of butter would give you the suggested daily intake of vitamin E (75mg).*

# How to take vitamins & minerals

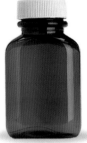

FOOD IS THE FIRST *source of vitamins and minerals. If you have an inadequate diet, or special needs, supplementation may be necessary. Modern stresses mean that our bodies often need more of particular nutrients in order to function in response to the demands placed upon them. A nutritionist will help you to analyze any deficiencies and decide with you the best form in which to take the supplements recommended.*

ABOVE **All supplements have different quantities of the active ingredients. Check the quantity and the dosage recommended.**

ABOVE **Folic acid is one of the B vitamins and is commonly prescribed during pregnancy. It is also thought it may protect against cancer.**

| **POWDERS** | **CAPSULES** | **LIQUIDS** | **TABLETS** |
|---|---|---|---|
| Many vitamins and minerals – such as vitamin C – come in this form. Powders provide you with extra potency, with no additives (useful for people with allergies). | These are convenient to take and easy to keep. Fat-soluble vitamins are normally taken in capsule form, but many contain vitamin and mineral powders which allow a higher potency. | These are appropriate for people who have difficulty swallowing tablets or capsules. Many children's formulas come in liquid form for easy administration. Liquids can be mixed with food or drinks. | Most vitamins and minerals come in tablet form, which is the most practical form, because they can be stored easily and keep for a long time. Check the label to see what is added in the form of binders or fillers, which are added to preserve or bulk out the active ingredient. |

LEFT **Zinc capsules may be used as a supplement to protect the immune system.**

# FORMS

Vitamins and minerals come in various different forms, and some may be more appropriate for certain people than for others. The easiest way to find out what is best for you is to experiment – a powder may be easier to take than a capsule or tablet, particularly for children or older people. Some liquids and oils may cause a reaction in susceptible individuals; if you find that is the case for you, try another form.

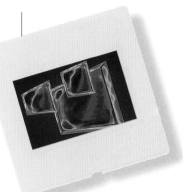

ABOVE **Crystals of vitamin A, which is one of the antioxidant vitamins. They boost immunity, fight cancer, and help to slow down the aging process.**

BELOW **Milk is a good source of vitamin D and calcium, both of which can help to prevent osteoporosis.**

## CHELATION

"Chelated" is a term which appears on mineral supplements. It means that the minerals are combined with amino acids to make assimilation more efficient. Use chelated products whenever possible because they are three to five times more effective.

## TIME-RELEASE

Time-release formulas allow them to be released into the body over an 8- to 10-hour period. These are useful for water-soluble vitamins, the excess of which is quickly excreted. Studies show that time-release formulas are very effective, providing stable levels.

## SYNTHETIC VITAMINS

Synthetic vitamins may cause toxic reactions, but natural vitamins won't. Natural vitamins are superior; synthetic vitamins will work, but they will never be as potent, or as free of side-effects, as the real thing.

# Key vitamins & minerals

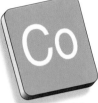

ABOVE **Minerals have a particular chemical composition which has its own notation; e.g. I for iodine and Co for cobalt.**

EVERY VITAMIN AND MINERAL *has its own specific properties and role within our bodies. By insuring that we have adequate quantities in our diets, we will be taking steps toward addressing any ailments we are currently suffering, as well as preventing future illness. Evidence also shows that vitamins and supplements can protect our bodies and reduce the risk of acquiring degenerative diseases. So the first step is to eat a varied, balanced diet, rich in the vitamins and minerals that are outlined in the subsequent pages of this book. The second step is to take a good multivitamin and mineral supplement, and perhaps add to your diet any nutrients which may have a therapeutic use.*

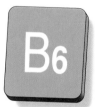

ABOVE **Vitamins are given letter and number names.**

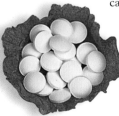

ABOVE AND RIGHT
*The current RDA for vitamin B12 is 1.5–2mcg, which is easily provided by 30g of mackerel. Capsules and tablets may contain between 10 and 100mcg.*

Governments around the world have provided guidelines for how much of each vitamin or mineral we need in our diets. These are called RDAs (recommended daily allowances) or RDIs (recommended daily intakes) and they apply to healthy individuals with a good, balanced diet. These levels are "adequate" intake, and do not reflect new thinking on nutrition for optimal health and longevity. In other words, they are not therapeutic levels and they do not take into account the varying needs of the population. People with illnesses, a stressful lifestyle, who are on medication, or who eat a highly refined diet, may need more than the RDA.

In the following pages, each vitamin and mineral is described, with natural

**US RDA**
recommended daily allowance in the US

**EU RDA**
recommended daily allowance in the EU

**EAR**
estimated average requirements

**WHO**
World Health Organization

**IU**
international units

**mg**
milligrams

**mcg**
micrograms

*Supplements: maximum safe dosage*

sources listed, along with the current RDA for the US and the European Union. Deficiency symptoms are also described, alongside the functions of the vitamin or mineral in our bodies. The therapeutic dosages which might be appropriate for certain conditions are also noted. If you plan to take large doses of vitamins or minerals, contact your physician or a nutritionist for advice.

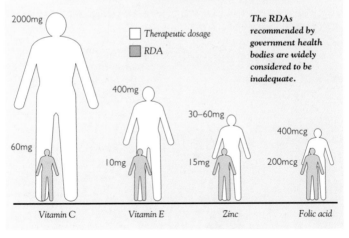

## RDA LEVEL VS SUPPLEMENT LEVEL

☐ *Therapeutic dosage*
▨ *RDA*

*The RDAs recommended by government health bodies are widely considered to be inadequate.*

| Vitamin C | Vitamin E | Zinc | Folic acid |
|---|---|---|---|
| 2000mg | 400mg | 30–60mg | 400mcg |
| 60mg | 10mg | 15mg | 200mcg |

# Vitamin A

*Boosts immunity*
●
*Treats disorders
of the skin*

**US RDA 5,000 IU**

**EU RDA 800mcg
(2,700 IU)**

*Some dosages as
high as 15,000 IU
(as retinol) but it is
not recommended
that pregnant
women have
any more than
5,000 IU per day.
Beta-carotene
is not toxic.*

*Vitamin A is a fat-soluble vitamin
which comes in two forms: retinol,
found in animal products like liver,
eggs, butter, and cod liver oil, and
beta-carotene, which our body converts
into vitamin A when we need more.*

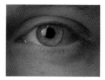

ABOVE **Vitamin A
improves night vision.**

Beta-carotene is
found in any
bright-colored fruits
and vegetables.

Vitamin A was for many years
called a "miracle" vitamin because
of its significant effect on the
immune system and its importance
for growth. It is necessary for
healthy skin and eyes, and lets us
see effectively in the dark. Beta-
carotene is an antioxidant
*(see page 13)*, and it also has
anticarcinogenic properties.

## FURTHER FUNCTIONS

- Anticarcinogenic
- Prevents aging of skin
- Improves vision and prevents night blindness
- Improves body's ability to heal
- Promotes growth of strong bones, hair, teeth, skin, gums
- May help in the treatment of hyperthyroidism

## DEFICIENCY SYMPTOMS

- Night blindness
- Persistent headaches
- Reduced resistance to infections (particularly respiratory)
- Skin problems
- Dry, brittle hair
- Kidney stones

## DOSAGE

- The RDA is believed to be inadequate, and people with special needs (following illness, for example), should have more
- As beta-carotene – doses up to 25,000 IU can be used to prevent illness. Do not exceed 15,000 IU as retinol

## TOXICITY

- Vitamin A as retinol is toxic and should not be taken at all by pregnant women. Beta-carotene is not toxic and is considered to be safe for adults and children alike

LEFT **Halibut liver
oil capsules are a rich
source of vitamin A.**

# Vitamin B1

B1

*Thiamin is involved in all key metabolic processes in the nervous system, heart, blood cells, and muscles.*

ABOVE **Vitamin B1 is found in all plant and animal foods.**

It is useful in the treatment of nervous disorders, and is singular in that it can protect against imbalances caused by alcoholism. There are more cases of vitamin B1 deficiency than of any other nutritional element – probably because of the high rate of alcoholism. Thiamin is found in all plant and animal foods, but good sources are whole grains, brown rice, seafood, and legumes. Vitamin B1 is essential for digestion and for the nervous system. Optimum intake of the vitamin will help us to cope with stress.

Helps to convert sugar to energy in the muscles and bones

•

Helps to treat heart disease

**US RDA**
1.2–1.5mg

**EU RDA** 1.4mg

*Supplements of 10–100mg are recommended; see below for special cases.*

BELOW **Brown rice is an excellent natural source of vitamin B1.**

## FURTHER FUNCTIONS

- Protects against imbalances caused by alcohol consumption
- May help in the treatment of neurological disease
- May help to treat anemia
- May improve mental agility

## DEFICIENCY SYMPTOMS

- Fatigue
- Muscle weakness
- Loss of appetite
- Irritability
- Depression
- Poor memory
- Tingling in the toes and soles of the feet
- Indigestion
- Nausea
- Beri-beri

## DOSAGE

- Heavy drinkers, smokers, pregnant women, or those taking the pill should increase normal dosage to up to 100–300mg per day
- Increase in stressful conditions. Most effective as part of a good B-complex supplement

## TOXICITY

- There are no reports of toxicity

# Vitamin B2

*Protects against cancer*

•

*Helps to promote growth*

•

*Promotes healthy skin and hair*

US RDA 1.7mg

EU RDA 1.6mg

*Supplements 10–300mg*

RIBOFLAVIN *is a water-soluble member of the B-complex family of vitamins.*

It is crucial to the production of body energy and has anti-oxidant qualities (*see page 13*). Riboflavin is not stored in any significant amount in the body, and deficiency is common. The best natural sources are milk, liver, kidneys, yeast, cheese, and leafy green vegetables.

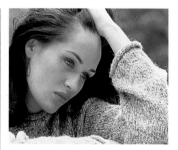

ABOVE *Vitamin B2 is essential for the body to produce energy; chronic fatigue may indicate a slight deficiency.*

## FURTHER FUNCTIONS

- Helps to metabolize fats, protein, and carbohydrates
- Aids vision
- Promotes healthy reproductive function
- Boosts athletic performance
- Protects against anemia

## DEFICIENCY SYMPTOMS

- Cracked skin and mucus membranes
- Reddening of the tongue
- Eczema of skin and genitals
- Burning sensation on skin
- Fatigue

## DOSAGE

- Pregnancy, breastfeeding, taking the pill, and heavy drinking all call for an increase in intake
- Take as part of a B-complex supplement, and increase dosage in stressful situations. 100–300mg are commonly suggested

## TOXICITY

- Toxic in very high doses; minor, rare symptoms include itching and burning of the skin

BELOW **Hard cheese is a rich source of riboflavin.**

# Vitamin B3

NIACIN *is one of the water-soluble B-complex vitamins, and it is essential for the synthesis of sex hormones and a healthy nervous system.*

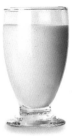

ABOVE
**Milk contains vitamin B3.**

Niacin may also help to prevent or cure schizophrenia, and act as a detoxificant, ridding the body of toxins, pollutants, and drugs. Niacin is found in liver, lean meats, whole grains, peanuts, eggs, avocados, and fish.

It takes the form of nicotinic acid and nicotinamide, and is a fairly recent addition to the family of B-complex vitamins, named as a vitamin in 1937.

*Promotes healthy digestion*

•

*May prevent migraine headaches*

•

*Reduces high blood pressure*

| US RDA |
|---|
| 13–18mg adults |
| 5–6mg infants |
| 9–13mg children under 10 |

| EU RDA |
|---|
| 15–18mg |
| *Supplements 20–100mg* |

LEFT **Avocados are rich in many vitamins.**

## FURTHER FUNCTIONS

• Prevents and treats schizophrenia
• Aids in cell respiration
• Produces energy from sugar, fat, and protein
• Maintains healthy skin, nerves, tongue, and digestion
• May lower cholesterol, and protect against heart disease

## DEFICIENCY SYMPTOMS

• Dermatitis
• Diarrhea
• Dementia, all of which are symptoms of pellagra (see page 9)

## DOSAGE

• Large doses may be used therapeutically, but should be taken under the supervision of a physician or practitioner
• Doses of 20–100mg of niacin, taken daily, may be beneficial. Best taken as part of a B-complex supplement

## TOXICITY

• Symptoms include depression, liver malfunction, flushing, and headaches in high doses
• Avoid doses larger than about 120mg unless you are under the supervision of a physician

# Vitamin B5

*Helps in the production of energy*
•
*Aids in the reduction of stress*
•
*Controls metabolism of fat*

**US RDA 10mg**
**EU RDA 6mg**
*Supplements up to 100mg*

PANTOTHENIC ACID *is a water-soluble member of the B-complex family of vitamins which helps to maintain normal growth and the health of the nervous system.*

Pantothenic acid has become a popular supplement over the past decade for its ability to boost energy levels and improve the immune response. There is also evidence that it can lower cholesterol and protect against heart disease. The best natural sources include meat, whole grains, bran, kidneys, nuts, chicken, molasses, and eggs.

Pantothenic acid is useful in reducing the effects of stress on the body.

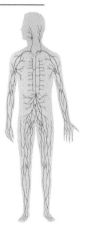

ABOVE *Vitamin B5 encourages the action of the lymphatic system which governs our immune response.*

## FURTHER FUNCTIONS

• Encourages healing of wounds
• Encourages the immune system
• Prevents fatigue
• Lowers cholesterol levels and protects against heart disease
• Prevents and treats arthritis

## DEFICIENCY SYMPTOMS

• Vomiting
• Cramps
• Fatigue
• Insomnia
• Reduced resistance to infection
• Abdominal pain

## DOSAGE

• Best taken in B-complex formulas, up to 300mg per day for therapeutic use
• Normal dosage, which should help to prevent illness, is about 100mg per day

RIGHT *Molasses – rich in vitamin B5.*

## TOXICITY

• No known toxicity; doses of over 300mg per day should be supervised by a practitioner

# Vitamin B6

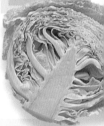

B6

*Helps prevents skin and nervous disorders*
•
*Eases nausea*

| | |
|---|---|
| **US RDA** | 2mg |
| **EU RDA** | 1.6–2mg |
| *Supplements* | *50–200mg* |

PYRIDOXINE *is a water-soluble B-complex vitamin which is necessary for the production of antibodies and white blood cells.*

B6 is necessary for vitamin B12 to be absorbed. B6 is required for the functioning of more than 60 enzymes in the body and is needed for protein synthesis. Of all the B-vitamins, B6 is the most important for a healthy immune system, and it is thought to protect the body against some cancers. B6 is widely used for the symptoms of PMS and the menopause, and may cure some forms of infertility. Natural sources include brewer's yeast, liver, kidneys, heart, melon, cabbage, molasses, and eggs.

RIGHT **Cabbage is a good source of vitamin B6.**

## FURTHER FUNCTIONS

- Boosts immunity
- Helps to control diabetes
- Assimilates proteins and fats
- Treats symptoms of PMS and menopause
- Reduces muscle cramps and spasms
- Acts as a natural diuretic
- Protects against cancer

## DEFICIENCY SYMPTOMS

- Anemia
- Nervous disorders
- Skin problems

## DOSAGE

- Should always be taken as part of a B-complex supplement, and in equal amounts with B1 and B2
- Time-release formulas are best because it lasts for only 8 hours in the body. Avoid intake of more than 50–200mg unless under the supervision of a professional

## TOXICITY

- Toxic in high doses, causing serious nerve damage when taken in quantities of more than 200mg per day

LEFT **B6 supplementation is common because many modern diets do not have adequate quantities.**

# Vitamin B12

*Promotes healthy growth in children*

•

*Increases energy levels*

**US RDA 3mcg (maximum absorbable quantity is 8mcg)**

**EU RDA 2mcg**

*Supplements 5–50mcg*

COBALAMIN *is a water-soluble member of the B-complex vitamin family, and it is the only vitamin that contains essential minerals.*

B12 is essential for a healthy metabolism of nerve tissue, and deficiencies can cause brain damage and neurological disorders. B12 may also reduce the risk of cancer and the severity of allergies, as well as boosting energy levels. B12 was once considered to be a "wonder drug" and was given by injection to rejuvenate.

Good sources include liver, beef, pork, eggs, cheese, and milk.

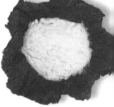

RIGHT **Vitamin B12 was the last true vitamin discovered, in 1948.**

| FURTHER FUNCTIONS | DEFICIENCY SYMPTOMS | DOSAGE | TOXICITY |
|---|---|---|---|
| • Necessary for maintenance of the nervous system<br>• Improves memory and concentration<br>• Required to utilize fats, carbohydrates, and proteins<br>• May protect against cancer<br>• Protects against allergens and toxic elements | • Pernicious anemia<br>• Menstrual problems<br>• Mental deterioration<br>• Trembling | • Dosages of between 5–50mcg should be adequate for most people; higher dosages should be supervised. Best taken as part of a B-complex supplement | • Not believed to be toxic<br><br>BELOW **Liver is a good source of vitamin B12.** |

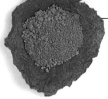

# Folic Acid

ABOVE **Taken early in pregnancy, folic acid can prevent spina bifida in the unborn baby.**

FOLIC ACID *is a water-soluble vitamin which forms part of the B-complex family. It is also known as vitamin Bc.*

*Necessary for the metabolism of RNA and DNA*

•

*Essential for blood formation*

**US RDA**
**400mcg**

**EU RDA**
**200–360mcg**

*Supplements 400–800mcg for pregnant women*

Recent findings indicate that folic acid can prevent some types of cancer and birth defects, and it is helpful in the treatment of heart disease. Folic acid is essential for the division of body cells, and is needed for the utilization of sugar and amino acids. Taken from just before conception, and particularly in the first trimester of pregnancy, folic acid can prevent spina bifida. Food sources include deep green leafy vegetables, carrots, yeasts, liver, whole grains, avocados, egg yolks, melon, and apricots, therefore folic acid deficiency is usually the result of a poor diet.

## FURTHER FUNCTIONS

- Improves lactation
- Improves skin
- Natural analgesic
- Increases appetite
- Builds up resistance to infection in infants
- Essential for genetic code transmission
- Prevents spina bifida

## DEFICIENCY SYMPTOMS

- Weakness
- Lethargy
- Extreme fatigue
- Sleeplessness
- Irritability
- Dementia
- Possibly spina bifida

RIGHT **Many varieties of legumes are an important source of folic acid in our diet.**

## DOSAGE

- There are many people at risk of deficiency, including heavy drinkers, pregnant women, the elderly, and those on low-fat diets. Supplementation at 400–800mcg is recommended for those at risk
- Best taken with a good multivitamin and mineral supplement

## TOXICITY

- Toxic in large doses and can cause severe neurological problems. Do not take if you have or suspect B12-deficiency anemia

# Vitamin C

*Boosts immunity*
•
*Fights cancer*

**US RDA
60mg**

**EU RDA 60mg**

*Supplements
up to 3,000mg
(1,500 is commonly
recommended)*

VITAMIN C *is taken by more people than any other supplement and yet studies show that a large percentage of the population have deficiencies.*

Vitamin C is also known as ascorbic acid, and it is one of the most versatile of the vitamins we need to sustain life. It is one of the antioxidant vitamins *(see page 13)* and is believed to boost immunity and to fight cancer and infection. Good sources include rosehips, blackcurrants, broccoli, citrus fruits, and all fresh fruits and vegetables. Vitamin C is water-soluble, which means that any excess is excreted in the urine.

RIGHT **Citrus
fruits are still the
best natural source
of vitamin C.**

| FURTHER FUNCTIONS | DEFICIENCY SYMPTOMS | DOSAGE | TOXICITY |
|---|---|---|---|
| • Antioxidant<br>• Speeds up healing of wounds<br>• Maintains healthy bones, teeth, and sex organs<br>• Acts as a natural antihistamine<br>• May help to overcome male infertility<br>• Reduces the duration of colds and other viruses | • Weakness<br>• Poor healing ability<br>• Irritability<br>• Bleeding gums<br>• Bruising easily<br>• Loose teeth<br>• Joint pain<br>• Scurvy | • At least 60mg is necessary for health, but more is required by smokers (25mg is depleted with every cigarette), and people suffering from stress or an infection, taking antibiotics, drinking heavily, or after an accident or injury | • May cause kidney stones and gout in some individuals. Some people suffer from diarrhea and cramps at high dosages<br><br>LEFT **Rosehips are rich in vitamin C and many supplements are produced from them.** |

30

# Vitamin D

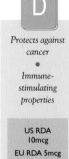

D

*Protects against cancer*

•

*Immune-stimulating properties*

VITAMIN D *is a fat-soluble vitamin which is found in foods of animal origin; it was isolated in 1930 from cod liver oil and is known as the sunshine vitamin.*

ABOVE **Sunlight is necessary for our bodies to synthesize vitamin D.**

**US RDA**
10mcg

**EU RDA 5mcg**

*Supplements*
*200–400 IU*
*(5–10mcg)*

Vitamin D can be produced in the skin from the energy of the sun, and it is not found in rich supply in any food. Vitamin D is important for calcium and phosphorus absorption, and helps to regulate calcium metabolism. Recent research suggests that it could have a role in protecting against some cancers and infectious diseases. Deficiency is caused by inadequate exposure to sunlight, and low consumption of foods containing vitamin D.

## FURTHER FUNCTIONS

- Protects against osteoporosis
- May help in the treatment of psoriasis
- Boosts the immune system
- May be useful in treatment of cancer
- Necessary for strong teeth and bones

## DEFICIENCY SYMPTOMS

- Rickets
- Osteomalacia
- Bone pain
- Muscular weakness and spasm
- Osteoporosis

## DOSAGE

- Supplementation between 200 and 400 IU is suggested for those at risk of deficiency
- Best taken as part of a good multivitamin and mineral supplement

## TOXICITY

- Vitamin D is the most toxic of all the vitamins, causing nausea, vomiting, headache, and depression, among other symptoms Do not take in excess of 1,000 IU daily

RIGHT **Vitamin D is found in mackerel, and all oily fish.**

# Vitamin E

*Boosts immunity*
•
*Alleviates fatigue*

**US RDA 30 IU**
**EU RDA 10mg**
*Supplements up to 800 IU*

VITAMIN E, *also known as tocopherol, is fat-soluble and one of the key antioxidant vitamins* (see page 13).

Apart from its crucial anti-oxidant value, vitamin E is important for the production of energy and the maintenance of health at every level. Unlike most fat-soluble vitamins, vitamin E is stored in the body for a short period of time, and up to 75 percent of daily doses are excreted in the feces. Its key function is as an anticoagulant, but its role in boosting the immune system and protecting against cardiovascular disease is becoming increasingly clear. Vitamin E is found in wheatgerm, soybeans, vegetable oils, broccoli, leafy green vegetables, whole grains, and eggs.

ABOVE *Fresh wheatgerm and wheatgerm oil are rich sources of vitamin E, but have little value if they are rancid.*

## FURTHER FUNCTIONS

• Antioxidant
• Protects against neurological disorders
• Protects against cardiovascular disease
• Reduces symptoms of PMS
• Treats skin problems
• Aids in the prevention of miscarriage

## DEFICIENCY SYMPTOMS

• None

BELOW *Vitamin E can be taken in tablet form by people who are sensitive to oil.*

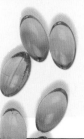

## DOSAGE

• Available in many forms (dry is best for people with skin problems or oil intolerance)
• Daily dosage may be 200–1,200 IU daily, but benefits can be obtained from daily doses of 30–400 IU
• Best taken with a good multivitamin and mineral preparation

## TOXICITY

• High doses may be toxic; take doses higher than 600 IU per day only under a physician's supervision

# Biotin

BIOTIN *is not a true vitamin, but it works with B-complex vitamins and is often called vitamin H, or co-enzyme R. Biotin is water-soluble and is found in many common foods.*

Essential for the
normal metabolism
of fat and protein
•
Helps maintain
healthy skin

**US RDA**
300mcg
**EU RDA**
0.15mg
*Supplements
25–300mcg*

Biotin is depleted in the body by alcohol, cooking or refining food, and antibiotics. Egg yolks are biotin-rich but raw egg whites contain avidin, a protein that prevents biotin absorption.

Biotin works more effectively with vitamins B2, B3, B6, and A.

Good sources include: nuts, fruits, beef, liver, egg yolks, milk, kidneys, unpolished rice, and brewer's yeast.

LEFT **Apples and
most other fruits
and vegetables
contain biotin.**

## FURTHER FUNCTIONS

• Prevents hair from graying
• Eases muscular aches and pains
• Treats eczema, dermatitis, and other skin conditions
• Helps to prevent baldness

## DEFICIENCY SYMPTOMS

• Eczema
• Fatigue
• Impairment of fat metabolism

## DOSAGE

• Biotin is normally included in most B-complex supplements, at 25–300mcg

## TOXICITY

• There are no known levels of toxicity

LEFT **Eczema
sufferers may be
wise to add
brewer's yeast and
egg yolks to their
diet; both are rich
in biotin, which
may prevent the
condition.**

# Boron

BORON *is a trace mineral found in most plants, and is essential for human health.*

Recent research has reported that boron added to the diets of post-menopausal women prevented calcium loss and bone demineralization – a revolutionary discovery for sufferers of osteoporosis. It is also claimed that boron will raise testosterone levels and build muscle in men, and is therefore often used by athletes and body builders. Boron is found in most fruit and vegetables, and does not appear in meat and meat products. Boron supplements are usually taken in the form of sodium borate.

*Beneficial in the treatment of arthritis*
•
*Prevents osteoporosis*
•
*Builds muscles*

| US RDA |
| no official figures |
| **EU RDA** |
| no official figures |
| **EAR 2mg** |
| *Supplements 1–3mg* |

ABOVE RIGHT
***Fruit is a source of boron.***

## FURTHER FUNCTIONS

• External treatment of bacterial and fungal infections

## DEFICIENCY SYMPTOMS

• Growth retardation
• Boron is associated with calcium, magnesium, and phosphorus metabolism
• Increased effects of stress on the body

RIGHT **Boron is present in most vegetables.**

## DOSAGE

• No RDA, 3mg used daily to prevent osteoporosis
• Best if taken with a good multivitamin and mineral supplement

## TOXICITY

• Toxic effects include: red rash, vomiting, diarrhea, reduced circulation, shock, and then coma
• Fatal dose is 15–20g, 3–6g in children. Symptoms appear at about 100mg

# Calcium

CALCIUM *is an important mineral, and recent research shows that we get only about one-third of what we need for good health.*

Calcium is essential for human life – it makes up bones and teeth, and is crucial to enable messages to be conducted along nerves. It ensures that our muscles contract and that our hearts beat, and it is extremely important in the maintenance of the immune system, among other things. There are many groups at risk of calcium deficiency – in particular, the elderly – and because it is so important to body processes, our bodies take what they need from our bones, which causes them to become thin and brittle.

Food sources include dairy produce, leafy green vegetables, salmon, canned sardines, and tofu.

*Works to create healthy bones and teeth*

•

*Promotes a healthy nervous system*

•

*Eases insomnia*

**US RDA**
**800–1,200mg**

**EU RDA 800mg**

*Supplements 200–1,000mg*

## FURTHER FUNCTIONS

- Treatment and prevention of osteoporosis
- Prevents cancer
- Helps to prevent heart disease
- Treats arthritis
- Keeps skin healthy
- Eases leg cramps
- Encourages heartbeat
- Helps the body to metabolize iron

## DEFICIENCY SYMPTOMS

- Rickets
- Osteoporosis
- Weak bones and teeth
- Leg cramps

## DOSAGE

- Experts recommend that calcium be taken in a good multivitamin and mineral supplement, although extra doses may be given up to 1,000mg per day

## TOXICITY

- Doses over 2,000mg per day may cause hypercalcemia, but excess calcium is excreted so that toxic dosage is unlikely

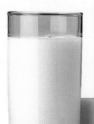

LEFT **Rich sources of calcium include milk and cheese.**

# Cobalt

**Co**

*Works with vitamin B12 in:*

•

*the production of red blood cells*

•

*the health of the nervous system*

| US RDA |
|---|
| no official figures |
| **EU RDA** |
| no official figures |
| **WHO** |
| recommends |
| 1 mcg |

*Not often supplemented other than with vitamin B12, but up to 30mg may be used*

COBALT *is an essential trace mineral which is a constituent of vitamin B12.*

The amount of cobalt you have in your body is dependent on the amount of cobalt in the soil, and therefore in the food we eat. Most of us are not deficient in cobalt, although deficiency is much more common in vegetarians. Foods that are rich in cobalt include fresh leafy green vegetables, meat, liver, milk, oysters, and clams.

RIGHT **Intakes of cobalt depend on the level in the soil, which affects the amount that plants and animals receive from it.**

## FURTHER FUNCTIONS

Cobalt can, with vitamin B12:
• prevent pernicious anemia
• aid in the synthesis of DNA and choline

## DEFICIENCY SYMPTOMS

• There are no specific deficiency symptoms of cobalt, but as a component of vitamin B12, anemia can result from an inadequate intake

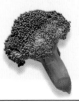

## DOSAGE

• Cobalt is rarely found in supplement form, but forms part of a good multivitamin and mineral supplement with the B-complex vitamins
No daily allowance set, but 8mcg is suggested as a necessary quantity in the diet

## TOXICITY

• When used therapeutically, side-effects occurred at doses above 30mg; these included goiter, hypothyroidism and heart failure

LEFT AND ABOVE
**Broccoli is a good source of cobalt if it is grown in cobalt-rich soil.**

# Chromium

CHROMIUM *is a trace mineral which was discovered to be important to our health in the 1950s. It is an important regulator of blood sugar, and has been used successfully in the control and treatment of diabetes. Studies into the functions of chromium are ongoing and promising.*

Treats and prevents diabetes

•

Helps in the treatment of hypoglycemia

•

Protects against heart disease

Good sources of chromium include whole grain cereals, meat, cheese, brewer's yeast, molasses, and egg yolk. Fruits and vegetables have a relatively small quantity and refined grain products have almost none.

BELOW **Wholewheat bread contains chromium, which helps control blood sugar levels.**

**US RDA**
no official figures

**EU RDA**
no official figures

*Supplements*
50–200mcg

| **FURTHER FUNCTIONS** | **DEFICIENCY SYMPTOMS** | **DOSAGE** | **TOXICITY** |
|---|---|---|---|
| • Aids in the control and production of insulin<br>• Aids in metabolism<br>• Controls blood cholesterol levels<br>• Stimulates the synthesis of proteins<br>• Increases resistance to infection | • May cause diabetes<br>• Nervous problems<br>• May cause some heart disease<br>• Associated with increased blood cholesterol and fat levels | • There is no RDA, but it is suggested that 25mcg per day is adequate<br>• Supplements up to 200mcg per day may be appropriate<br>• Take as part of a good multivitamin and mineral supplement | • Less than 10 percent of chromium taken by the body is absorbed, so there is very little chance of toxicity |

LEFT **The metal chromium is extracted from the mineral chromite.**

# Copper

**Protects against cardiovascular disease**

•

**Useful in the treatment of arthritis**

**US RDA 1.5–3mg**

**EU RDA 1.2mg**

*Supplements 1.5–3mg*

COPPER *is an essential trace mineral and is necessary for the act of respiration – iron and copper are required for oxygen to be synthesized in the red blood cells.*

Copper is also important for the production of collagen, which is responsible for the health of our bones, cartilage, and skin. Copper is also one of the antioxidant minerals *(see page 13)*, which protect against free-radical damage.

Food sources of copper include animal livers, shellfish, nuts, fruit, oysters, kidneys, and legumes.

RIGHT *A copper deficiency can cause brittle bones and supplements are often provided to sufferers of osteoporosis.*

| FURTHER FUNCTIONS | DEFICIENCY SYMPTOMS | DOSAGE | TOXICITY |
|---|---|---|---|
| • May help to prevent cancer<br>• Boosts the immune system<br>• Acts as an antioxidant | • Anemia<br>• Edema<br>• Brittle bones<br>• Irritability<br>• Loss of sense of taste | • Supplementation can lower the levels of zinc in the body and cause insomnia, so care should be taken<br>• A copper bracelet worn against the skin allows some copper to be absorbed<br>• Copper appears in good multivitamin and mineral supplements | • Excess intake can cause vomiting, diarrhea, muscular pain, and dementia, but toxicity is low<br>• Can be taken in doses up to 3mg |

LEFT *Good natural sources include most shellfish.*

# Fluorine

FLUORINE *is a trace mineral found naturally in soil, water, plants, and animal tissues. Its electrically charged form is "fluoride," which is how we usually refer to it.*

*Protects against tooth decay*
•
*Protects against osteoporosis*

**US RDA**
1mg fluoride
3.6mg sodium fluoride

**EU RDA**
No official figures but most people get 1mg from water

*Supplements up to 10mg are all right, where the water is not fluoridated*

Although it has not yet been officially recognized as an essential nutrient, studies show that it is important in many processes, and may play a major role in the prevention of many twentieth-century killers, like heart disease.

LEFT **Most toothpastes contain fluoride, which protects against decay.**

The main source of fluorine is drinking water, which is often artificially fluoridated. Foods high in fluoride include seafood, animal meat, and tea. Fluoride supplements should always be taken with calcium.

## FURTHER FUNCTIONS

• May help to prevent heart disease
• May help to prevent calcification of organs and musculoskeletal structures

## DEFICIENCY SYMPTOMS

• May cause infertility or anemia, although this link is still being investigated
• Tooth decay
• Osteoporosis

## DOSAGE

• Major source is drinking water, and typical daily intake is 1–2mg. Tablets and drops are available from pharmacies, but should be limited to 1mg daily in adults, and 0.25–0.5mg for children. Do not supplement fluoride without the advice of your dentist

## TOXICITY

• Fluorosis causes irregular patches on the enamel, and depresses the appetite. Eventually the spine calcifies. Fluorosis is rare and occurs at levels far above 10mg per day

LEFT **Drinking water will have fluoride added to it unless there is enough occurring naturally.**

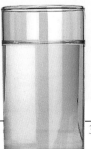

# Iron

*Prevents and cures iron-deficiency anemia*

•

*Improves immunity*

**US RDA**
10–18mg
(30mg for pregnant women)

**EU RDA** 14mg

*Supplements 5–25mg*

IRON *is a trace mineral which is essential for human health. Iron-deficiency anemia, which is the condition most commonly associated with severe shortage of the mineral, was described by Egyptian physicists as long ago as 1500* B.C.

Today we know that iron is present in our bodies as hemoglobin, which is the red pigment of blood. Iron is required for muscle protein and is stored in the liver, spleen, bone-marrow, and muscles. Food

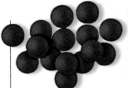

LEFT *Iron supplementation on its own should only be undertaken upon the advice of your physician or a health professional.*

sources include shellfish, brewer's yeast, wheatbran, offal, cocoa powder, dried fruits, and cereals.

| **FURTHER FUNCTIONS** | **DEFICIENCY SYMPTOMS** | **DOSAGE** | **TOXICITY** |
|---|---|---|---|
| • Improves physical performance <br> • Anticarcinogenic <br> • Prevents learning problems in children <br> • Boosts energy levels | • Anemia <br> • Pallor <br> • Tiredness <br> • Breathlessness <br> • Insomnia <br> • Palpitations | • Pregnant, breastfeeding, and menstruating women, infants, children, athletes, and vegetarians may require increased levels of iron. Iron supplements will be prescribed by your physician if necessary <br> • Maximum dosage is 15mg daily, unless under supervision | • Excess iron can cause constipation, diarrhea, and rarely, in high doses, death |

RIGHT *Parsley and other leafy green vegetables such as spinach are rich in iron.*

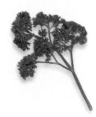

# Germanium

GERMANIUM *is a mineral which is abundant in the surface of the earth.*

There is no sound evidence that it is essential to human life, but recent studies indicate that many conditions respond favorably to therapeutic doses of germanium. Germanium is believed to function by boosting the action of oxygen in generating energy, and because it maintains equilibrium within the body, it is said to reduce high blood pressure, lower cholesterol levels, and exert a good effect on the immune system. Germanium is now considered to be one of the antioxidant minerals *(see page 13)*.

RIGHT **Many medicinal herbs, including comfrey, ginseng, and garlic, are rich sources of germanium.**

*Considered antioxidant*

•

*Stimulates the immune system*

**US RDA**
no official figures

**EU RDA**
no official figures

*Supplements up to 10g seem safe but 25–500mg best*

## FURTHER FUNCTIONS

• Useful in the treatment of cancer
• Protects against osteoporosis
• May be analgesic
• May have antiviral, antibacterial, and antitumor activity

## DEFICIENCY SYMPTOMS

• Possibly reduced immune activity but this has not been confirmed

## DOSAGE

• Germanium supplementation is not recommended without a physician's supervision
• Good multi-vitamin and mineral supplements will contain an acceptable level of germanium

## TOXICITY

• Germanium is safe up to quite a high level, although skin eruptions and diarrhea were reported in some patients taking therapeutic doses

# Iodine

IODINE *is a mineral which was first discovered in 1812 in kelp. It was extracted and named iodine because of its violet color,* ion *being Greek for violet.*

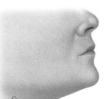

Iodine occurs naturally and is a crucial part of the thyroid hormones which monitor our energy levels. Iodine is found in seafood and seaweeds, and most table salt is fortified with iodine. Anyone who eats large quantities of cruciferous vegetables should consider an iodine supplement.

Thyroid
cartilage

Thyroid gland

RIGHT **Our body concentrates iodine in the thyroid gland situated at the base of the neck. Iodine is necessary for thyroid function.**

## FURTHER FUNCTIONS

- Relieves pain of fibrocystic breasts
- Protects against toxic effects from radioactive materials
- Prevents goiter
- Acts as a natural antiseptic

## DEFICIENCY SYMPTOMS

- Goiter
- Hypothyroidism, which causes chronic fatigue, apathy, dry skin, intolerance to cold, weight gain, and thyroid enlargement

## DOSAGE

- Best taken as potassium iodide
- Take under the supervision of your physician or nutritionist. 150mcg per day RDA is adequate

## TOXICITY

- Iodine is toxic in high doses and may aggravate or cause acne. Large doses may interfere with hormone activity

LEFT **Haddock and other white fish are, along with kelp and seaweed, the richest natural sources of iodine.**

# Potassium

POTASSIUM *is one of the most important minerals in our bodies, working with sodium and chloride and other important substances to form "electrolytes," or the essential electrically charged ions which make up our bodily fluids.*

weakness
muscle pains

Normalizes blood pressure

Involved in most important functions in our bodies

US RDA
900mg

EU RDA 3,500mg

*Supplements rare, is rich in foods*

ABOVE *Potassium deficiency can cause muscular problems, and make us tire easily.*

Potassium is crucial for body functioning, playing a role in nerve conduction, our heartbeat, energy production, synthesis of nucleic acids and proteins, and muscle contraction. Potassium can be found in fresh fruit and vegetables – in particular, bananas. Sweating causes a loss of potassium, as does chronic diarrhea and diuretics.

## FURTHER FUNCTIONS

- Maintains water balance within cells
- Stabilizes internal structure of cells
- Helps to conduct nerve impulses
- May protect against stroke
- Improves athletic performance
- May help treat and prevent cancer

## DEFICIENCY SYMPTOMS

- Vomiting
- Muscular weakness and paralysis
- Muscle pains
- Overwhelming fatigue
- Low blood pressure

## DOSAGE

- Eat more fresh fruit and vegetables to increase potassium intake. Diuretic users and those in a hot climate may need up to 1.5g daily
- Take with zinc and magnesium

RIGHT *Raisins are a good source of potassium (880mcg per 100mg).*

## TOXICITY

- May cause muscular weakness and mental apathy, eventually stopping the heart. May cause ulceration of the small intestine

# Magnesium

*Protects against cardiovascular disease*

•

*Helps to treat Pre-menstrual Syndrome (PMS)*

**US RDA**
**300–400mg**

**EU RDA 300mg**

*Supplements 200–500mg*

MAGNESIUM *is a mineral which is absolutely essential for every biochemical process in our bodies, including metabolism and the synthesis of nucleic acids and protein.*

Magnesium deficiency is very common, particularly in the elderly, heavy drinkers, pregnant women, and regular, strenuous exercisers, and it has been proved that even a very slight deficiency can cause a disruption of the heartbeat. Good sources of magnesium are brown rice, soybeans, nuts, brewer's yeast, wholewheat flour and legumes.

RIGHT **Magnesium may be used for problems of the nervous system.**

## FURTHER FUNCTIONS

- Helps to prevent kidney and gallstones
- Useful in treatment of high blood pressure
- Useful in treatment of prostate problems
- Repairs and maintains body cells
- Required for hormonal activity

## DEFICIENCY SYMPTOMS

- Weakness
- Tiredness
- Nervous convulsions and behavior
- Unsteadiness
- Hyperactivity in children
- Low blood sugar
- Palpitations

## DOSAGE

- Dietary intake is thought to be inadequate in the average Western diet; supplements of 200–500mg are recommended daily
- Good multi-vitamin and mineral supplements should have a healthy dose of magnesium

## TOXICITY

- Magnesium is toxic to people with renal problems or atrioventricular blocks. Other than these cases, magnesium should be safe

LEFT **Whole grains are a good source; the refining process leaves white bread with little or no magnesium.**

# Manganese

MANGANESE *is an essential trace element which is necessary for the normal functioning of the brain, and is effective in the treatment of many nervous disorders, including Alzheimer's disease and schizophrenia.*

*Necessary for the functioning of the brain*

•

*Used in the treatment of some nervous disorders*

Our understanding of manganese is still incomplete, but it may prove to be one of the most important nutrients in human pathology. It is likely that manganese is one of the antioxidant minerals *(see page 13)*. Sources include cereals, tea, green leaf vegetables, wholewheat bread, legumes, and nuts.

| US RDA |
|---|
| 2.5–7mg |
| EU RDA |
| no official figures |
| *Supplements* |
| *2–10mg* |

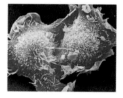

LEFT **Manganese is necessary for the repair and maintenance of all body cells.**

## FURTHER FUNCTIONS

- Necessary for normal bone structure
- Important in the formation of thyroxin
- Necessary for reproduction
- Necessary for glucose metabolism

## DEFICIENCY SYMPTOMS

- Fatigue
- Poor memory
- Nervous irritability
- Ataxia
- Related to diabetes, heart disease, and rheumatoid arthritis

## DOSAGE

- Best taken in a good multivitamin and mineral supplement
- 2–5mg is considered adequate, but doses up to 10mg are thought to be safe

## TOXICITY

- Very rare, but may include lethargy, involuntary movements, posture problems, and coma. Environmental toxicity may be possible

RIGHT **Legumes are a good dietary source of manganese.**

# Molybdenum

Protects against
cancer

•

Protects teeth
against tooth decay

MOLYBDENUM *is an essential trace element, and a vital part of the enzyme which is responsible for the utilization of iron in our bodies.*

**US RDA**
150–500mcg

**EU RDA**
no official figures

*Supplements
50–100mcg*

RIGHT **Molybdenum
can prevent sexual
impotence in men
and is necessary
for a healthy
reproductive system.**

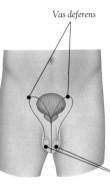

Vas deferens

Testes

Molybdenum may also be an antioxidant (*see page 13*), and recent research indicates that it is necessary for optimum health. Best food sources include wheat, canned beans, wheatgerm, liver, legumes, whole grains, offal, and eggs. Molybdenum can help to prevent anemia and is known to promote a feeling of well-being.

## FURTHER FUNCTIONS

• Aids in the metabolism of fats and carbohydrates
• Vital for the utilization of iron in our bodies
• Prevents anemia
• Prevents sexual impotence

## DEFICIENCY SYMPTOMS

• Irregular heartbeat
• Inability to produce uric acid
• Irritability

## DOSAGE

• The optimal intake is still undecided; adequate amounts are between 7.5 and 25mcg per day, but intake will differ between individuals. Experts suggest 50–100mcg per day to prevent ill health

RIGHT **Buckwheat is
an excellent natural
source of molybdenum.**

## TOXICITY

• Molybdenum is toxic in doses higher than 10–15mg, which cause gout-like symptoms

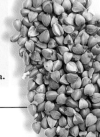

# Phosphorus

PHOSPHORUS *is a mineral which is essential to the structure and function of the body.*

*Increases endurance and energy levels*

•

*Reduces fatigue and creates a sense of wellbeing*

**US RDA
800–1,200mg**

**EU RDA 800mg**

*Supplements
1,000mg*

ABOVE **Foods rich in phosphorus include milk, canned fish, and nuts; excess quantities will throw off mineral balance and decrease calcium levels.**

It is present in the body as phosphates, and in this form aids the process of bone mineralization and helps to create the structure of the bone. Phosphorus is also essential for communication between cells and energy production. Phosphorus appears in many foods – in particular, yeast products, wheatgerm, hard cheeses, canned fish, nuts, cereals, and eggs.

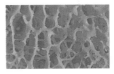

LEFT **The human bone requires phosphorus for normal structure and function.**

| **FURTHER FUNCTIONS** | **DEFICIENCY SYMPTOMS** | **DOSAGE** | **TOXICITY** |
|---|---|---|---|
| • Forms bones and teeth<br>• Burns sugar for energy<br>• Acts as a co-factor for many enzymes and activates B-complex vitamins<br>• Forms RNA and DNA | • Weakness<br>• Bone and joint pain<br>• General debility<br>• Loss of appetite<br>• Irritability<br>• Neurological symptoms<br>• Speech problems<br>• Mental confusion<br>• Anemia<br>• Lowered resistance to infection | • Phosphorus deficiency usually accompanies deficiency in potassium, magnesium, and zinc, so take a good multivitamin and mineral supplement with all four<br>• Supplementation should only be undertaken with supervision | May occur with dosages or intake above 1,000mg per day. May cause:<br>• diarrhea<br>• calcification of organs and soft tissues<br>• prevention of iron, calcium, magnesium, and zinc absorption |

# Selenium

Acts as an antioxidant and may discourage the aging process

•

Stimulates the immune system

**US RDA**
50–100mcg

**EU RDA**
10–75mcg

*Supplements 50–200mcg with vitamin E*

RIGHT **The name selenium is derived from the moon goddess Selene.**

SELENIUM *is an essential trace element which has recently been recognized as one of the most important nutrients in our diet.*

ABOVE **Kidneys provide the richest source of dietary selenium (about 40mg per 100g).**

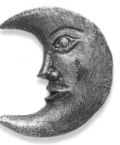

It is an antioxidant (*see page 13*), and is vitally important in human metabolism. Selenium has been proved to provide protection against a number of cancers and other diseases. Best sources of selenium include wheatgerm, bran, tuna fish, onions, tomatoes, broccoli, kidneys, and wholewheat bread.

## FURTHER FUNCTIONS

• Prevents many cancers
• Maintains healthy eyes and eyesight
• Maintains healthy skin and hair
• Protects against heart and circulatory diseases
• Can detoxify alcohol, many drugs, smoke, and some fats
• Increases male potency and sex drive

## DEFICIENCY SYMPTOMS

• No specific symptoms, but deficiency can be the result of diets which are high in refined and processed foods

## DOSAGE

• It has been suggested that men take 75mcg of supplementary selenium, and women take 60mcg
• Dosages of 400–1,000mcg have been used for immune stimulation and for anti-carcinogenic effects, but 50–200mcg may be adequate

## TOXICITY

• Toxic in large doses; beware of blackened fingernails or garlic odor on skin and breath
• Daily intake should not exceed 450mcg unless supervised

# Silicon

SILICON *is a trace element which is only just becoming understood. It has been proved essential to animals and it is believed that silicon is as crucial to human life.*

Si

*Protects against some heart disease*

•

*Likely to play a role in metabolism of tissue, bone, skin, and fingernails*

**US RDA**
no official figures

**EU RDA**
no official figures

*Not usually a supplement on its own; take as part of a good general supplement*

I t is thought that silicon plays a part in the make-up of our connective tissues, bones, skin, and fingernails. Food sources include whole grains, vegetables, hard drinking water, and seafood. It is available as a supplement in the form of silicon dioxide. Silicea is also a popular homeopathic remedy.

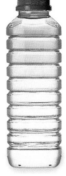

LEFT **Hard drinking water should supply adequate levels of silicon.**

| FUNCTION | DEFICIENCY SYMPTOMS | DOSAGE | TOXICITY |
|---|---|---|---|
| • Believed to help prevent hair loss<br>• May prevent osteoporosis by helping the body utilize calcium in the bones | • Unknown, but weakened nails, brittle bones and hair, and poor skin may be symptoms<br><br>RIGHT **Root vegetables, in particular potatoes, are rich in silicon which is the second most abundant element on earth.** | • There is no official RDA, but we need between 20 and 30mg each day. It is believed that we get about 200mg in our diet<br>• Supplementation best taken in the form of a multi-vitamin and mineral tablet; natural supplements contain up to 400mg | • Toxic if inhaled. Silicon in our food unlikely to be toxic<br>• May contribute to kidney stones |

# Vanadium

VANADIUM *is a trace mineral which has only recently been proved necessary for human life.*

At the turn of the century, French doctors believed that vanadium was a miracle cure for a variety of illnesses, but it proved to be toxic at the levels they were prescribing; not surprisingly, its popularity waned. Today, it is believed that elevated levels of vanadium may cause manic depression, which is perhaps a clue to a little understood disease. Vanadium is found in Seafood.

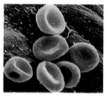

RIGHT **It is believed that vanadium may help the body to produce red blood cells.**

## FURTHER FUNCTIONS

Little is known for certain, but it is believed that it may:
• reduce high blood sugar
• help to prevent tooth decay
• aid in the production of red blood cells
• encourage normal tissue growth and fat metabolism

## DEFICIENCY SYMPTOMS

• None known, although diets with high levels of vitamin C are said to reduce the levels of vanadium in the body

RIGHT **Apart from parsley, lobster is the best-known source of vanadium.**

## DOSAGE

• Supplements are not available, although some of the newer multi-vitamin and mineral supplements may contain low levels of this element

## TOXICITY

• Vanadium is very toxic and is linked to manic depression in high quantities

# Zinc

Zn

**ZINC** *is one of the most important trace elements in our diet, and it is required for more than 200 enzyme activities within the body.*

ABOVE **It has now been proved that it is the zinc in oysters which increases male libido.**

It is the principal protector of the immune system, and is crucial in the regulation of our genetic information. Zinc is also essential for the structure and function of cell membranes. Zinc is an antioxidant *(see page 13)* and is found in offal, meat, mushrooms, oysters, eggs, whole grain products, and brewer's yeast. Zinc has recently been used in the treatment of rheumatoid arthritis, and may help to prevent the degenerative effects of aging.

*Boosts immune system*
•
*Prevents cancer*
•
*Prevents and treats the common cold*

US RDA
15mg

EU RDA
15mg

*Supplements*
*15–30mg*

## FUNCTION

• Prevents blindness associated with aging
• Increases male potency and sex drive
• Treats and prevents infertility
• Maintains senses of taste, smell, and vision
• Prevents hair loss
• Treats acne and other skin problems

## DEFICIENCY SYMPTOMS

• Poor appetite
• Growth retardation
• Lethargy
• Abnormal taste, smell, and vision
• Increased susceptibility to infections
• Underfunctioning sex glands
• Slow healing of wounds

## DOSAGE

• Take with a good multivitamin and mineral supplement. Daily, 15–30mg is useful; increase copper and selenium intake if taking more zinc

RIGHT **Zinc supplementation is suggested for a wide range of health conditions – from infertility to immune problems.**

## TOXICITY

• Zinc is thought to be nontoxic, although very high doses (above 150mg per day) may cause some nausea, vomiting, and diarrhea

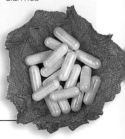

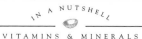
# Home use

IT MAY BE DIFFICULT *to pinpoint which vitamins and minerals are missing from your diet, and if you suffer from any long-term illnesses or are on medication, it is probably best to seek advice from a professional.*

There are a few tips to bear in mind when you are choosing which supplements to take:

• Avoid taking any one vitamin or mineral in large quantities, unless you are under the supervision of your physician or nutrition specialist.

• A good multivitamin and mineral supplement should cover all your needs, unless you are suffering from a specific condition which may warrant the use of particular nutrients.

• Eat a balanced diet and remember that supplements are not a replacement for food and they will not work without it.

• Take supplements regularly throughout the day, and with food (*see page 13* for exceptions).

• Extra doses of specific nutrients should not need to be taken for longer than 4 to 6 weeks, unless there are special circumstances. You should start to see results within 2 to 3 weeks of beginning supplementation. If not, the chances are that it is not doing any good.

Consult your doctor before beginning vitamin and mineral supplementation if you are:

• pregnant
• breastfeeding
• taking medication
• under the age of 12

LEFT *Supplements are no replacement for a balanced diet and healthy lifestyle.*

# Common ailments

THE FOLLOWING *conditions may respond to increased levels of some nutritional elements. This advice in no way replaces that of a physician or health practitioner, and before using supplements you should consider seeking expert attention. Never take more than the recommended dose noted on your supplement packaging unless it has been prescribed by a professional.*

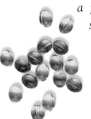

### ACNE

Try a multivitamin and mineral supplement which is low in iodine.
Increase intake of:
• Vitamin E (p.32)
• Vitamin A (p.22), as retinol, (see warning on page 22)
• Zinc (p.51)
Eliminate processed foods.

### ALLERGIES

Increase your intake of:
• Vitamin B12 (p.28)
• Vitamin C (p.30), which may improve the body's response to allergens.
Supplements to boost the immune system will help.

### ANEMIA

Increase your intake of:
• Iron (p.40)
• Vitamin B1 (p.23), B2 (p.24), and B6 (p.27)
• Vitamin C (p.30), between meals
• Folic acid (p.29)

### ARTERIOSCLEROSIS

Increase your intake of:
• B-complex vitamins (pp.23–9)
• Vitamins A (p.22) (as beta-carotene), C (p.30), and E (p.32)
• Selenium (p.48), magnesium (p.44), manganese (p.45), and zinc (p.51).
Reduce fats and processed foods in the diet.

## ARTHRITIS

Increase your intake of:
- Vitamins A (*p.22*), C (*p.30*), and E (*p.32*)
- B-complex vitamins (*pp.23–9*), 100mg, 3 times daily
- Vitamin D (*p.31*)
- Calcium (*p.35*) and magnesium (*p.44*), which are needed to form the fluid around the joints
- Copper (*p.38*), taken orally or worn as a bracelet
- Vitamin B5 (*p.26*), which proves useful in some cases

## ASTHMA

Increase your intake of:
- Vitamin C (*p.30*) (beware, because it can interfere with the medication you are taking; discuss treatment with your doctor)
- Vitamins A (*p.22*), B2 (*p.24*), B5 (*p.26*), B6 (*p.27*), and E (*p.32*) (in a dry form)

## COLDS

Increase your intake of:
- Vitamin C (*p.30*) (up to 2g per day during a cold)
- Vitamin A (*p.22*)
- Vitamin E (*p.32*)
- Selenium (*p.48*)
- Zinc (*p.51*)

## COLD SORES

Increase your intake of:
- Vitamin C (*p.30*) (time-release)

- Vitamin E (*p.32*), in oil taken internally and applied to the affected area
- Vitamin B1 (*p.23*)
- Zinc (*p.51*), to boost the immune system

## CONSTIPATION

- Chronic constipation may respond to an increased intake of B-complex vitamins (*pp.23–9*), particularly if it follows a course of antibiotics. Vitamin B1 is most effective. Increase your fiber intake.

## COUGHS

Increase your intake of:
- B-complex vitamins (*pp.23–9*)
- Vitamin C (*p.30*)
- Vitamin A (*p.22*) (as beta-carotene)
- Vitamin E (*p.32*)
- Selenium (*p.48*)
- Zinc (*p.51*) (all of which will boost immune activity)

## DANDRUFF

Increase your intake of:
- Selenium (*p.48*)
- Vitamin E (*p.32*)
- Vitamin C (*p.30*)
- B-complex vitamins (*pp.23–9*)
- Zinc (*p.51*)

## DEPRESSION

Increase your intake of:
- B-vitamins (*pp.23–9*), which address the nervous system

- Vitamin C (*p.30*)
- Vitamin E (*p.32*)
- Zinc (*p.51*)
- Magnesium (*p.44*)
- Calcium (*p.35*)

### DIABETES 🐿

Increase your intake of:
- Chromium (*p.37*)
- Potassium (*p.43*)
- Zinc (*p.51*) (chelated)
- B-complex vitamins (*pp.23–9*)

### DIARRHEA 🐿

Increase your intake of:
- Potassium, which is easily lost in diarrhea and vomiting
- Vitamins B1 (*p.23*) and B3 (*p.25*), which will address the digestive system
- Water, to flush the system.

Take a good multivitamin and mineral supplement with food when you are able to eat properly again, to replace lost nutrients.

### ECZEMA 🐿

Increase your intake of:
- Vitamin A (*p.22*) (as beta-carotene)
- B-complex vitamins (*pp.23–9*), particularly B2 (*p.24*) and B6 (*p.27*)
- Vitamin C (*p.30*)
- Zinc (*p.51*)

- Vitamin E (*p.32*)
- Biotin (*p.33*)
- Copper (*p.38*)

### FATIGUE 🐿

Increase your intake of:
- Calcium (*p.35*)
- Zinc (*p.51*)
- Magnesium (*p.44*)
(a combined deficiency can cause fatigue)
- Iron (*p.40*), if you suspect anemia
- Vitamins B6 (*p.27*) and B12 (*p.28*) for energy

### GLANDULAR FEVER 🐿

Increase your intake of:
- Vitamin C (*p.30*)
- Vitamin A (*p.22*)
- Vitamin E (*p.32*)
- Zinc (*p.51*)
- Magnesium (*p.44*)
- B-complex vitamins (*pp.23–9*)
(all of which will address the immune system)

### GOUT 🐿

Increase your intake of:
- Magnesium (*p.44*)
- B6 (*p.27*) and B12 (*p.28*), which act as mild diuretics and aid kidney function
- Molybdenum (*p.46*), as part of a good multivitamin and mineral supplement

**HAIR LOSS** ❧

Increase your intake of:
• B-complex vitamins (*pp.23–9*), high dosage tablet, twice daily
• Choline
• Inositol
• Calcium (*p.35*)
• Magnesium (*p.44*)
• Vitamins and minerals in a good multi-supplement

**HANGOVER** ❧

• Take a B-complex tablet (*pp.23–9*) before drinking, one while you are drinking, and one before bed.
• Take a good multivitamin and mineral tablet before bed. Make sure it contains biotin and selenium.
• If you have a hangover, take one B-complex tablet (*pp.23–9*), and one multivitamin and mineral tablet, twice daily until symptoms are eased.

**HAY FEVER** ❧

Increase your intake of:
• B-complex vitamins (*pp.23–9*), high dosage, 3 times daily
• Vitamin C (*p.30*), up to 2g daily

• Zinc (*p.51*)
• Selenium (*p.48*)
• Vitamins and minerals in a good supplement

**HEADACHES** ❧

Increase your intake of:
• Niacin (Vitamin B3) (*p.25*)
• B-complex vitamins (*pp.23–9*), preferably time-release capsules
• Calcium (*p.35*)
• Magnesium (*p.44*)

**HIGH BLOOD PRESSURE** ❧

Increase your intake of:
• Potassium (*p.43*) (discuss this treatment with your doctor as it can conflict with other medication)
• B-complex vitamins (*pp.23–9*)
• Calcium (*p.35*)
• Vitamin E (*p.32*)

**INFLUENZA** ❧

Increase your intake of:
• Vitamin C (*p.30*), at the first sign of flu
• Zinc (*p.51*)
• B-complex vitamins (*pp.23–9*)
• Vitamins A (*p.22*) and E (*p.32*)

### INSOMNIA

Take one calcium (*p.35*) and one magnesium (*p.44*) tablet just before bedtime (chelated if you can get it, *see page 19*).
Then increase intake of:
• Vitamin B6 (*p.27*)
• Vitamin B3 (*p.25*)
• Dietary calcium (*p.35*)

### ME

Increase your intake of:
• Vitamins and minerals which boost the immune response, including selenium (*p.48*), zinc (*p.51*), vitamin C (*p.30*), vitamin E (*p.32*), vitamins B5 (*p.26*) and B6 (*p.27*)
Insure you have an adequate intake of:
• Trace elements, which may be linked to the condition

### MENOPAUSAL SYMPTOMS

Increase your intake of:
• Vitamin E (*p.32*), which can ease headaches and hot flushes
• Vitamin B6 (*p.27*)
• Vitamin C (*p.30*)
• Iron (*p.40*)
• Calcium (*p.35*)
• Vitamin D (*p.31*)
• B-complex vitamins (*pp.23–9*)

### MENSTRUAL PROBLEMS

Increase your intake of:
• Vitamin B6 (*p.27*), up to 150mg, 3 times daily
• B-complex vitamins (*pp.23–9*)
• B12 (*p.28*), up to 150mg, 3 times daily
• Iron (*p.40*), as part of a good multivitamin and mineral supplement
• Magnesium (*p.44*)

### NAUSEA

• Take vitamin B6 (*p.27*) for morning sickness (consult your doctor first) and for travel sickness – appropriate for children in half doses.

### PMS (PRE-MENSTRUAL SYNDROME)

Increase your intake of:
• Vitamin B6 (*p.27*) up to 100mg, 3 times daily
• B-complex vitamins (*pp.23–9*)
• Vitamin E (*p.32*), preferably in dry form
• B12 (*p.28*), up to 100mg, 3 times daily
• Magnesium (*p.44*)
• Calcium (*p.35*)

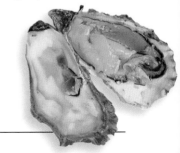

### PSORIASIS

Increase your intake of:
• Vitamin A (*p.22*), as beta-carotene
• Vitamin C (*p.30*)
• Vitamin E (*p.32*)
• Selenium (*p.48*)
• B-complex vitamins (*pp.23–9*) as part of a good multivitamin and mineral supplement
• Protein

### STRESS

• Take a good multivitamin and mineral supplement, with special attention to extra B-complex vitamins (*pp.23–9*) and vitamin C (*p.30*), which can be taken in extra doses.
• Take vitamin E (*p.32*) to 400 IU daily.

### THRUSH

Increase your intake of:
• Vitamins and minerals which improve immune activity (insure that all supplements are yeast-free):
• Vitamin C (*p.30*)
• Vitamin E (*p.32*)
• Vitamin A (*p.22*)
• Vitamin B-complex (*pp.23–9*)
• Selenium (*p.48*)
• Zinc (*p.51*)

### VARICOSE VEINS

Increase your intake of vitamins and minerals which improve circulation, including:
• Vitamin C (*p.30*)
• Vitamin E (*p.32*)
• Boron (*p.34*)
• Selenium (*p.48*)
• Silicon (*p.49*)

# Further reading

*Ruth Adams*, THE COMPLETE HOME GUIDE TO ALL THE VITAMINS (Larchmont Books, 1972)

*Martin Ebon*, WHICH VITAMINS DO YOU NEED? (Bantam Books, 1974)

*Leslie and Susannah Kenton*, RAW ENERGY (Arrow Books, 1991)

*Leonard Mervyn*, THORSONS COMPLETE GUIDE TO VITAMINS AND MINERALS (Thorsons, 1995)

*Earl Mindell*, THE VITAMIN BIBLE (Arlington Books, 1986)

*Hasnain Walji*, HEALTH ESSENTIALS : VITAMIN GUIDE (*Element Books, 1992*)

# Useful addresses

**The Council for Nutrition Education and Therapy (CNEAT)**
1 The Close
Halton, Aylesbury
Buckinghamshire HP22 5NJ

**Dietary Therapy Society**
33 Priory Gardens
London N6 5QU
0181 341 7260

**Health Education Authority**
Hamilton House, Mabledon Place
London WC1H 9TX

**Institute of Optimum Nutrition**
5 Jerdan Place, Fulham
London SW6 1BE

**Society for the Promotion of Nutritional Therapy**
PO Box 47, Heathfield
East Sussex TN21 8ZX
01435 867007
(Send an sae plus £1 for a copy of the register)

**American Association of Nutrition Consultants**
1641 East Sunset Road
Apt. B-117, Las Vegas
NV 89119 USA
1 709 361 1132

**American College of Advancement in Medicine**
PO Box 3427, Laguna Hills ,
CA 92654 USA

**American College of Nutrition**
722 Robert E. Lee Drive
Wilmington
NC 20927 USA

**American Dietetics Association**
216 West Jackson Boulevard
Apt. 800, Chicago
IL 60606–6995 USA
1 800 877 1600